Meal Prep

A Complete Meal Prep Cookbook with 30 Days Meal Plan for Weight Loss and 27+ Easy Recipes

The information in the following pages is broadly considered a truthful and accurate account of facts. As such, any inattention, use, or misuse of the information in question by the reader will render any resulting actions solely under their purview. There are no scenarios in which the publisher or the original author of this work can be in any fashion deemed liable for any hardship or damages that may befall them after undertaking information described herein.

Table of Contents

Introduction 1

Chapter 1: The Basics 5

Understanding Calories 5

Weight Loss Myths...7

How weight loss work 10

Prep Tips For Your Weight Loss Journey 11

Chapter 2: On Mindful Eating and Curbing Hunger 16

The Do's... 17

The Don'ts 20

The Do's...23

The Don'ts 25

Chapter 3: Recipes 28

Breakfast: Egg and Spinach Bowl (4 points)...............30

Lunch: Plant-based Borscht (2 points) 32

Dinner: Broccoli and Beef Stir Fry (7 points) 35

Breakfast: Hot Chocolate Oatmeal (6 points).............38

Lunch: Taco Lettuce Boats (3 points) 41

Dinner: Roast Beef with Side Salad (11 points)...........44

Breakfast: Soufflé Omelet with Mushrooms (1 point) .48

Lunch: Eggplant Parmesan Sandwich (8 points) 50

Dinner: Smoked Salmon with Egg Salad (1 point) 54

Breakfast: Blueberry Oat Pancakes (12 points)...........57

Lunch: Instant Pot Creamy Spaghetti (10 points) 60

Dinner: Slow Cooker Chicken Enchiladas (9 points)...63

Breakfast: Dairy Free Crepes (5 points) 66

Lunch: Chicken and Spinach Ramen Bowl (5 points) .69

Dinner: Creamy Chicken and Mushrooms (2 points)..72

Breakfast: Avocado Stuffed Deviled Eggs (1 points)....75

Lunch: Spinach and Mozzarella Frittata (3 points) 77

Dinner: Squash Gnocchi and Sage Butter Sauce (10 points) 80

Breakfast: Peach Pie Breakfast Parfait (10 points) 83

Lunch: French Onion Soup Casserole (7 points) 85

Dinner: BBQ Chicken and Avocado Quesadillas (9 points) 87

Breakfast: Gingerbread Pancakes (3 points)................89

Lunch: Pita Pocket Breakfast Sandwich (6 points)......92

Dinner: Southwest Veggie Wraps (6 points)................95

Breakfast: Ham and Poached Egg Muffin (6 points)...98

Lunch: Instant Pot Macaroni and Cheese (13 points)100

Dinner: Bean and Potato Soup (8 points) 102

Breakfast: Sweet Potato Breakfast Hash (6 points)...105

Lunch: Instant Pot Jambalaya (7 points)...................108

Dinner: Crispy Zucchini Tacos (8 points) 112

Breakfast: Baked Peanut Butter Banana Oatmeal (11 points) 116

Lunch: Black Bean and Sweet Potato Wrap (13 points) 118

Dinner: Caprese Pasta (12 points) 121

Breakfast: Three Seed Berry Parfait (6 points) 123

Lunch: Mediterranean Quinoa Bowl (5 points) 125

Dinner: Shrimp Stir-Fry (1 points) 127

Breakfast: Honey Nut Breakfast Cereal (8 points) 130

Dinner: Baked Chicken and Vegetable Spring Rolls (3 points) 134

Breakfast: Crustless Vegetable Quiche (2 points)...... 138

Lunch: White Chicken Enchiladas (12 points)............141

Dinner: Chicken and Broccoli Stir Fry (8 points) 144

Chapter 4: 30-day Meal Plan 148

Week 1: 149

Week 2: 151

Week 3: 152

Week 4: 153

Chapter 5: Grocery Buying Guide 156

Conclusion 161

Bonus Content 163

Introduction

Leading a healthier lifestyle is a goal for many people. Many of us want to make positive changes in our lives, but often find it difficult to do so due to different reasons. It may be not we tend to settle for what's convenient; to make our lives easier, despite knowing that doing so is also ruining our health. How many times have we chosen fast food or take out over cooking something for dinner? Just because food from your favorite take out place looks healthy, it doesn't always mean that it is.

But it isn't just the need for convenience that's putting our health at risk. There's also we fail to recognize and change bad eating habits that we have developed. We eat mindlessly, often distractedly. In front of the TV, while working, and even whilst moving from one place to another. We try our best to eat as quickly as possible; failing to savor our food. Then, we wonder why we feel so hungry again just an hour or so after devouring a meal. It's because many of us aren't able to eat mindfully.

These are just two of the things that we'll be tackling in this book—as part of the Weight Loss Program. More than just dieting, we'll do our best to help set you on the path towards a lifestyle change. One that you can easily sustain and maintain. This is among the principles of the Weight Loss and Meal Prep program, after all. More than just dieting, it's about giving people the right tools to help them make better choices for their health.

In this book, you'll find:

- Tips and techniques for eating mindfully.

- 27+ delicious and healthy recipes meant to help you lose weight, whilst also making sure you enjoy your meals.

- A 30-Day Meal Prep program, to help you get a feel for what the process is like and enable you to seamlessly integrate it into your lifestyle.

Remember, it isn't about breaking habits. It often comes down to making better ones that will replace the old ones that were holding you back.

We wish you the best with your weight loss and health journey!

CHAPTER 1

The Basics

Most people believe that slow metabolism is the culprit behind obesity. Some may point to age, poor diet that has too much meat or sweets and various other reasons. Yes, those factors may contribute to weight gain, but they're not the main cause.

So, why do people gain weight? The answer is simple; they consume too much calories.

Understanding Calories

Calories, which are obtained through the food and drinks that you consume, are the fuel the body uses to function normally.

Every movement, whether it's the beating of your heart or the twitch of your muscles, burns calories. The process in which your body converts food to energy is called metabolism.

The problem occurs when you take in more than you can burn. Your body stores the excess calories and converts them to fat. Repeat the process several times and you end up a few pounds heavier than you should be.

Weight loss occurs when you burn more calories than you consume – otherwise known as weight loss deficit.

There are other factors at play here as well. For example, if you have more muscle mass, you have higher basal metabolic rate – the rate at which your body uses up energy when you're at rest. This means that you are more likely to quickly burn calories.

So you see, it's even more important to maintain fitness so you can enjoy food without worrying too much about gaining weight.

Weight Loss Myths

There are a lot of myths concerning weight loss, and a lot of individuals have taken them as fact, though the opposite may be true. Some of these myths are:

α. **Fasting is the fastest way**

This is a very dangerous weight loss regime if you don't know what you're doing. Not only are you making yourself suffer, you're also cutting off your body's nutrient supply. You are more likely to have hunger pangs, which can cause binge eating later on the day. It's a very hard process to maintain and can lead to nutrient deficiencies. You're probably not even losing fat at all, and are shedding water and muscle mass instead. If you have to try fasting, you need to know what you're doing. Intermittent fasting in particular is one effective method that won't harm you when done right.

β. **Low-fat foods are a must-eat when dieting**

Low fat or sugar doesn't necessarily mean low-calories. In fact, low-fat food tends to contain more sugar than its regular counterparts. Sugar is dangerous because it's the kind of energy source that quickly gets stored as body fat when ingested but not burned off.

χ. **Exercising is enough**

While exercise is great for a weight loss program, it wouldn't make much difference if eat more than you can burn. Planning your meals is just as important as exercise.

δ. **Dieting is enough**

If you watch what you eat, you can lose weight. However, to ensure that your weight loss is sustainable, you have to ingrain some form of physical activity into your daily life. Dieting alone is good, but the results can be better if you add in some exercise.

ε. **Getting rid of carbohydrates in your diet is vital**

This is not always true because not all carbohydrates are bad. Simple carbohydrates such as sweets and candies can be excluded from your diet, as they provide empty calories and no nutritional value. Complex carbohydrates such as whole wheat bread, however, should still be included.

How weight loss work

To truly lose weight, you simply have to create a calorie deficit.

Basically, you have to eat less than your Basal Metabolic Rate, which is the number of calories your body burns per day.

Let's say your BMR is 2,000 calories a day. One pound of fat is equivalent to 3,500 calories, so if you aim to lose two pounds you'll have to cut 500 calories off your food intake. Your calorie limit will be 1500 kcal per day for the next 14 days.

You can use calculators online to get the ideal calorie limits for your body and weight loss goals.

It's tempting to raise the number to a thousand a day to lose weight faster, but remember that your body needs those calories. It's best to stick to at least 300 and at most 500 calorie deficits per day to avoid drawbacks. Remember that you are trying to lose weight, not starve.

Prep Tips For Your Weight Loss Journey

Right before we dive in to the losing weight segment, there are some things to remember. Think of it as pre-diet phase. Just as you need to warm up before you participate in rigorous exercise, you need to prepare your body for the changes in your diet.

📁🖐 Buy weight tracking equipment

You don't need to shell out too much money for fancy equipment, just one measuring tape, a notebook or journal, and a weighing scale will do. Measure your waist and weigh yourself, then jot all these numbers down, along with the date, to a journal or notebook. Do this before you start the program and continue doing so every week or two during your meal plan to see your progress. A reminder: don't be discouraged if you see little to no progress at first. These kind of changes take time.

📄🖋 **Watch your calories, but be kind to yourself**

There will be days when you'll be tempted to eat outside of your meal regime. Whether it's a single piece of cookie or a chocolate bar after lunch, you need to know how much extra calories you've eaten so you can try to burn it off with some physical activity. Don't worry; it doesn't need to be an intense workout. Just a jog up and down the stairs or a brisk 5-minute walk around your yard will be enough, depending on the calories you have to burn. Don't stop trying just because you gave in once. It will be easier eventually.

A calorie counter will also come in handy, you can download one as an app on your phone, or you can simply search it on the internet.

▤🖎 **Be ready to adjust your sleeping pattern**

If you sleep really late and wake up at 11 AM every morning, it's time to shift your sleeping schedule. This is to make sure you're awake early enough to prepare and eat your breakfast. If you find it hard, change it gradually. Sleep 30 minutes earlier each night until you've found your perfect sleeping pattern.

Tell your loved ones about your meal plan

This is to make sure that your friends and family know what you can and cannot eat. Their support can be uplifting if you're starting to falter. You can also look to online weight loss support groups and communities for encouragement and motivation.

CHAPTER 2

On Mindful Eating and Curbing Hunger

Switching to a healthier lifestyle, especially after you've been used to doing things a particular way for so long will take some adjustment. There will be challenges and you might find yourself falling behind at certain points—understand that this is totally fine. What matters is that you get back on track, exert a bit more effort, and make some necessary changes that will support the kind of life you want to have.

When it comes to eating healthier, it's more than just selecting the right food and doing portion control. Your overall mental approach matters just as much and being mindful about how you do things can really help make things easier. With that said, here are a few Do's and Don'ts to keep in mind.

The Do's

- Do start with your shopping list.

Always take your time and make sure you feel focused when writing your list. Mindfulness is key when it comes to creating the right grocery list that will benefit your goals. Think about how you've been feeling lately—what does your body require at the moment? With that in mind, start putting together your choices and edit it as you go.

- Do savor your meals.

Here's the thing, most people actually rush through their meals because of various reasons. Some may not have a lot of time to spare, whilst there are those who want to use that time for something else "more important". However, it is important to relish your food; take the time to enjoy its flavor, its aroma, and chew properly. Eating mindfully also makes you feel sated for a longer period of time.

- Do the "mouth full, hands empty" mantra.

This means that you should set your cutlery down in between mouthfuls of food. Quite similar to the previous tip, this is meant to help slow your eating and enable you to better appreciate your food. Not only that, doing this can actually help increase the response of your gut peptides. You'll feel full for longer and keep you from overeating.

- Always wait a minute or two before going back for seconds.

This allows the food you just ate to settle down and give you enough time to think if you really want more. Most people have a tendency to immediately go for seconds right after eating, especially if the food is something they really like. However, this often leads to them feeling too full and bloated. So, take your time after finishing your plate. Have some water or a sip of tea, then decide if you really need to refill your plate.

- Do keep your bigger serving bowls of food off the table and out of sight.

This is to serve the previous step's purpose. If you cannot immediately see or reach the food, you won't be able to refill your plate quickly. It also keeps you from craving more just because you keep seeing food. As you may or may not know, just the mere visual of delicious food can make us overeat. If we can see it and smell even while eating, we're bound to grab more servings.

The Don'ts

- Don't eat while you're distracted by something.

A lot of us fall into the trap of multi-tasking; in this case, eating whilst doing something else. Maybe you do it while you're watching TV, while you're working, or while you're moving from one place to the next. Sure, it feels good to be accomplishing a lot of things at the same time, but did you know that this can be detrimental to your fitness goals? By doing this, you're likelier to overeat or end up snacking again later. This is because your brain isn't fully processing the fact that you're eating.

So next time, give yourself an hour or 30 minutes to eat your meals.

- Don't drink too much alcohol before you begin eating.

Aside from its calorie content, research has shown that people who drink more before eating are actually more prone to cheating on their diets. Alcohol is also known to stimulate are appetites, making it harder for us to say no to food we cannot have.

- Don't eat when you're feeling stressed.

A lot of us have a tendency to "eat our feelings" as a means of relieving stress or any emotional distress we may be experiencing. Whilst this does seem to work, it can also cause us to overeat and feel guilty later on. Instead of turning to food during stressful moments, try mindfulness meditation instead. This will help turn our attention away from what we're craving (usually very indulgent food items) and is also a healthier alternative to stress eating.

- Don't forego your diet just because you're eating out.

As we've already established, there are ways of still following your diet even when you're out with friends. Remember, people also tend to eat more when they're in social settings or surrounded by friends. Don't stress yourself out when the menu for an event or a restaurant does not fit into your WW freestyle diet. Where you might not be able to be pickier of what you eat, you can always opt for portion sizes.

Eating mindfully is one thing, but the real challenge often happens when you're trying to beat hunger. It can make just about anyone restless and even cranky—everyone's familiar with this. Here are a few do's and don'ts to keep in mind when it comes to curbing your hunger:

The Do's

- Do your best to always get enough sleep.

Not getting enough sleep actually affects the balance of your hormones related to the appetite. Research shows that people who have had less than 5 hours of sleep experienced an increase in the ghrelin levels in their body. This is the hormone which actually triggers appetite and decreases leptin levels. Leptin is the hormone that signals our brain when we've had enough food.

- Do a bit of cardio after eating.

Doing this has a positive effect on our satiety hormones, helping promote a longer feeling of satiety. Research also proves that doing moderate-intensity exercises can curb feelings of hunger. It is also an effective form of distraction, keeping you from unintentionally eating or snacking.

When you start feeling the need to snack, try going for a walk instead. After you get back from it, you're bound to feel less inclined to grab a bag of chips or snack on your favorite treats. Note that the brain actually enjoys when we form new habits so do try and focus on making healthier ones, instead of trying to break your current bad habits. You'll eventually replace them when the good habits stick.

- Do have a hearty breakfast.

Breakfast is important—essential to our day. Having a hearty one provides our body with the ample fuel it needs to give you a head start on the day. People who begin their day with a protein-rich breakfast are less likely to begin craving snacks halfway through their morning. It also keeps you from overeating when lunchtime comes around, effectively preventing body fat gain and enabling you to manage your hunger better.

The Don'ts

- Don't eat too many fatty foods.

Having too much dietary fat in your daily meals can actually trigger ghrelin, the hunger hormone. Basically, the fattier the food you eat is, the greater your appetite for it would become. Just think back to all the times you've eaten food like French fries, pizzas, steaks, and so on—it's usually really hard to stop, right? This is why.

Another thing to pay attention to is your low-fat food's total energy content. These type of food is likely to contain great amounts of sugar to compensate for any flavor that's lost due to the low-fat content.

- Don't deprive yourself of your favorite foods.

It's totally okay to enjoy the foods you love, but make sure you do so moderately. Doing so actually helps you deal with cravings better and makes you feel less guilty about having them as well. Banning a food only serves to increase your craving for it so don't be afraid to have your favorites whenever you really feel like them.

CHAPTER 3

Recipes

Planning your meals isn't exactly the easiest, but it is also one of the most fun parts of Weight loss. If you're the type to experiment, here is where you can introduce foods you've been wanting to try. It also pushes you to be more creative with what you make, using recipes that are as simple or as complicated as you want them to be.

These are meals that can be easily achieved by beginners, working individuals, and even families who are looking to introduce healthier yet delicious foods to their everyday menu.

Note that every recipe comes with its value in Freestyle SmartPoints (Weight Watchers) so you can easily budget your everyday menu. I've also include important nutritional facts, so you know exactly what you're putting into your body. Lastly, remember that the points point to a single serving of the dish. If you're to go for seconds, multiply your total count by two.

Happy eating!

Breakfast: Egg and Spinach Bowl (4 points)

Yield: 4 servings

Nutritional info: calories 84, saturated fat: 1g, total fat: 2g, cholesterol: 57, trans fat: 0g, carbs: 6g, dietary fiber: 1g, sodium: 335mg, protein: 11g, sugar: 2g

Ingredients:

- 1 whole egg

- 8 egg whites

- 1 cup chopped or torn baby spinach

- ¼ cup feta cheese

- ½ cup diced tomatoes

- Sea salt

- ½ teaspoon black pepper

Directions:

➢ Preheat you oven to 350 degrees.

➢ Whisk all the ingredients together then lightly mist 4 ramekins with non-stick cooking spray. Separate your egg mixture equally into each one.

➢ Place your ramekins atop a cookie sheet the bake until eggs puff up. This should take around 20 minutes.

➢ Serve hot.

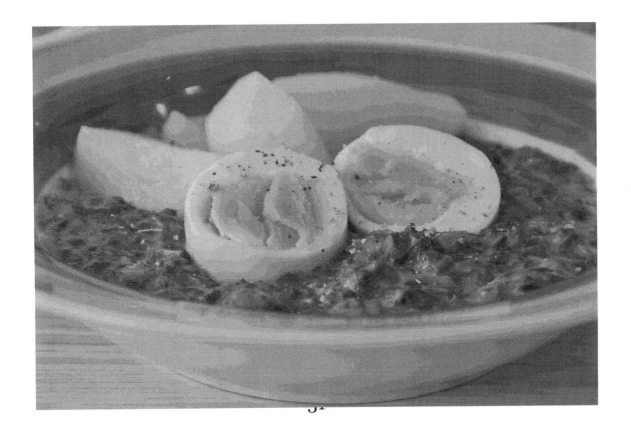

Lunch: Plant-based Borscht (2 points)

Yield: 6 cups

Nutritional Info: calories: 78, saturated fat: 0g, total fat: 1g, trans fat: 0g, sodium: 79mg, cholesterol: 0mg, carbs: 17g, sugar: 8g, fiber: 4g, protein: 3g

Ingredients:

(Borscht)

- ½ pound celery root

- 1 large carrot

- 1 medium zucchini

- 1 medium red onion

- ½ large red bell pepper

- 1 medium tomato

- 6 ounces red cabbage

- 2 medium beets

- 1 lemon

- 3 cups vegetable broth; prepare extra for liquid sauté

- ¼ cup fresh parsley

- Salt and pepper

(Tofu sour cream, an optional addition)

- 1 tablespoon lemon juice

- 1 extra film silken tofu

- 1 tablespoon red wine vinegar

- Salt and pepper

Directions:

- ➢ Peel and wash the veggies. Next, grate the zucchini, carrots, beets, and red cabbage.

- ➢ Chop the tomato, onion, and bell pepper into cubes.

- ➢ Liquid sauté the vegetables for 3 to 5 minutes.

- ➢ Heat another 3 cups of broth in a large pot until it boils. Reduce to a simmer.

- ➢ Add sautéed vegetables to the broth and simmer for 25 minutes. Add salt and pepper for taste.

- ➢ Squeeze 1 lemon into the broth.

Tofu Sour Cream

- ➢ Puree all the ingredients until smooth.

- ➢ Chill before serving.

- ➢ Leftovers will keep for 2 weeks in the fridge.

Dinner: Broccoli and Beef Stir Fry (7 points)

Yield: 4

Nutritional Info: calories: 206.1, total fat: 10.4g, saturated fat: 2.3g, sodium: 61.6mg, cholesterol: 60mg, carbs 2.8g, protein: 21g, sugar: 2.2g, dietary fiber: 1.5g

Ingredients:

- Lean flank steak, 12oz

- Broccoli, 3 cups of small florets

- Dry or sweet sherry, 2tbsp

- Ginger root, 2tbsp minced

- Cornstarch

- Low sodium soy sauce

- Peanut oil, 2tbsp divided

- Table salt, ½ tsp divided

- Onion, ½ cups sliced thinly

- Hoisin sauce, 2tbsp

- Sriracha chili sauce, 3tbsp

Directions:

➢ Boil 4 cups of water. Add the broccoli and cook for 1 minute. Drain.

➢ Cut beef into ¼ inch thick slices. Next, combine the meat with 1 tablespoon of sherry, ginger, soy sauce, ¼ teaspoon of salt, and cornstarch. Mix in 1 teaspoon of oil. In a different bowl, mix the rest of the ingredients.

➤ In a skillet, add 1 tablespoon of peanut oil and onions. Cook until fragrant then set aside. Next, cook the beef for 1 minute. Mix onions and beef until lightly browned.

➤ Add the rest of the oil to the skillet, toss in broccoli, then sprinkle the rest of the salt. Swirl in the sriracha and stir fry for another minute until veggies are crisp.

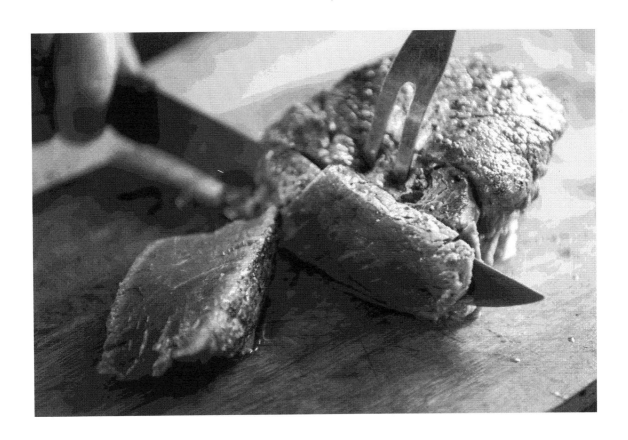

Breakfast: Hot Chocolate Oatmeal (6 points)

Yield: 4 servings

Nutritional Info: calories: 126, saturated fat: 6.4g, total fat: 8g, trans fat: 0g, sodium: 160mg, cholesterol: 0mg, carbs: 12.4g, sugar: 4.4g, dietary fiber: 2.1g, protein: 2.7g

Ingredients:

- 1 cup steel cut oats

- ½ cup coconut milk

- 4 cups water

- 1 teaspoon vanilla

- ¼ teaspoon salt

- 1 teaspoon cocoa powder

- 8 drops liquid stevia

- 1 teaspoon coconut palm sugar

Directions:

➤ Combine water, vanilla, milk, and stevia in a large bowl. Whisk in the sugar, cocoa, and salt.

➤ Next, stir in the oats. Oil the inside of the slow cooker so it doesn't stick. Pour the mixture in.

➤ Set cooker to low for 1 to 2 hours. Keep warm before leaving it.

➤ Top with shaved dark chocolate.

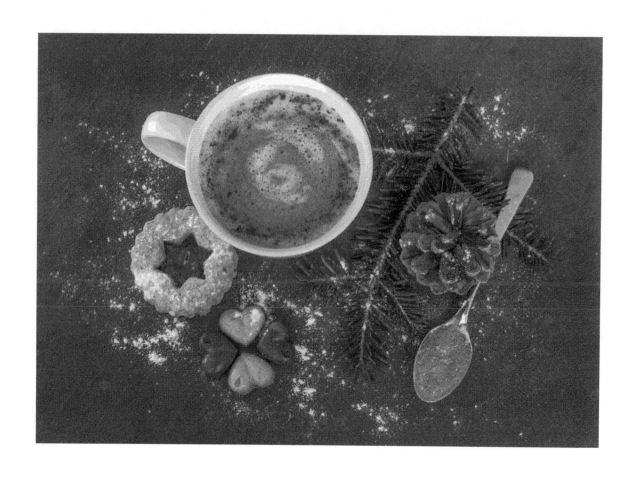

Lunch: Taco Lettuce Boats (3 points)

Yield: 6 servings

Nutritional Info: calories: 97, saturated fat: 2g, total fat: 5g, trans fat: 0g, sodium: 138mg, cholesterol: 10mg, carbs: 9g, sugar: 3g, dietary fiber: 2g, protein: 4g

<u>Ingredients:</u>

- 2 tablespoons extra virgin olive oil

- 1 medium onion, minced and separated

- 1 garlic clove

- 11 ounces ground lean turkey

- 1 cup tomatoes, finely chopped and separated

- 1 tablespoon soy sauce

- Ground pepper

- ½ teaspoon salt

- 6 lettuce leaves, washed and dried

- Finely chopped chives (optional)

- 1/3 cup low fat cheese, grated

Directions:

➢ Add extra virgin olive oil to a saucepan then sauté half of the onions with the garlic.

➢ Add half of the tomatoes in after a minute.

➢ Add the turkey and season this with salt, pepper, and soy sauce.

➢ Toss until it cooks thoroughly.

➤ Use the lettuce as bowls and even distribute the turkey atop. Add the remaining onions, cheese, and tomato. Top with chives.

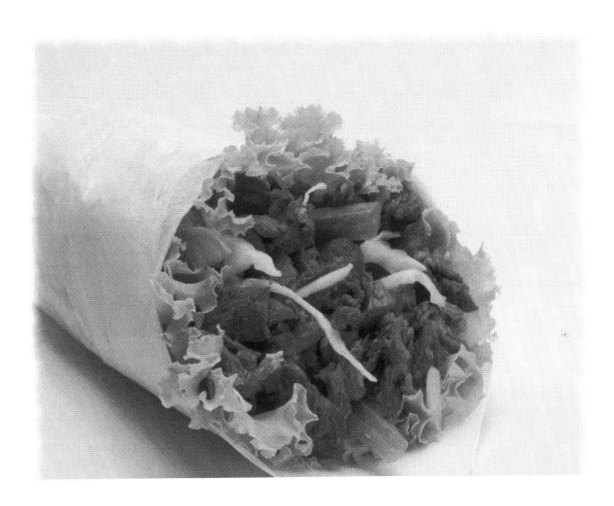

Dinner: Roast Beef with Side Salad (11 points)

Yield: 4 servings

Nutritional Facts: calories: 319, saturated fat: 5g, total fat: 18g, trans fat: 0g, carbs: 22g, sodium: 299mg, sugar: 16g, fiber: 3g, protein: 19g.

Ingredients:

(Roast beef)

- 4 portions of cooked lean roast beef. Leftovers can be used for this.

- 2 teaspoons of extra virgin olive oil

- 1 to 2 teaspoons of horseradish

- 1 tablespoon soy sauce

(Salad with raspberry vinaigrette)

- Salad greens mix of your choice

- 1 ½ tablespoons of extra virgin olive oil

- 1 tablespoon red wine vinegar

- 2 teaspoons honey

- 1 teaspoon Dijon mustard

- 2 tablespoons raspberries

- 1 pinch black pepper

- ¼ teaspoon sea salt

Directions:

(Salad)

➤ Puree the raspberries with the honey, vinegar, salt, pepper, and mustard. Switch to the lowest speed and drizzle in olive oil.

➤ Drizzle this over the greens or serve on the side.

(Roast beef)

➤ Whisk horseradish into soy sauce.

➤ Add 2 teaspoons of olive oil into a pan over medium heat. Add the beef and soy sauce. Cook for 2 minutes, stirring every now and then, until it is heated thoroughly.

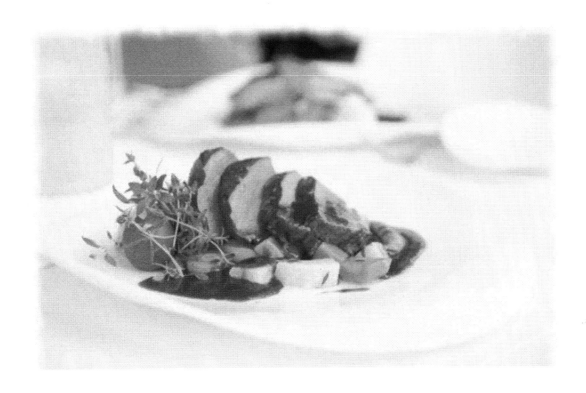

Breakfast: Soufflé Omelet with Mushrooms (1 point)

Yield: 6 servings

Nutritional Facts: calories: 72, saturated fat: 2g, total fat: 5g, trans fat: 0g, fiber: 0g, carbs: 2g, protein: 6g, sugar: 1g, sodium: 162mg, cholesterol: 98mg

Ingredients:

- 1 teaspoon of extra virgin olive oil

- 8 ounces of sliced mushrooms

- 1 garlic clove

- 3 large eggs

- 1 tablespoon of parsley, minced

- ½ teaspoon of pepper

- ½ teaspoon of salt

- ¼ cup of cheese, grated

Directions:

➤ Warm olive oil and sauté garlic. Add the mushrooms and sauté for another 10 minutes. Add the parsley then set aside.

➤ Whisk egg yolks. Next, beat the whites until frothy. Fold the whites in with the yolks, season with salt and pepper, then add cheese.

➤ Use non-stick spray on a large skillet.

➤ Pour in the egg mixture then cook until both top and bottom has set.

➢ Loosen the omelet then add the mushrooms before folding it.

➢ Serve hot.

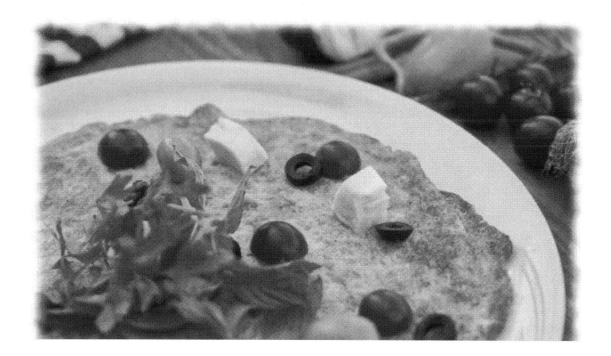

Lunch: Eggplant Parmesan Sandwich (8 points)

Yield: 12 servings

Nutritional Facts: calories: 300, saturated fat: 2g, total fat: 5g, carbs: 52g, protein: 13g, sugar: 6g, fiber: 6g, sodium: 610mg, cholesterol: 11mg

Ingredients:

- 2 egg whites

- 1 eggplant sliced into ¼ thick half-moon pieces

- 2 cups whole wheat panko bread crumbs

- 1 teaspoon salt

- 6 whole wheat ciabatta rolls, halved

- 1 cup fat-free mozzarella, shredded

- 1 ½ cups no-sugar marinara sauce, hot

- ¼ cup fat-free parmesan, grated

Directions:

➢ Preheat the oven to 400 degrees.

➢ Sprinkle salt on the eggplant and set aside for 10 minutes. This will make it softer. Rinse and dry after.

➢ Gently whip the egg whites. Dip each slice of the eggplant into this, then again into the panko. Coat all side evenly.

➢ Place the pieces on a baking sheet and bake for 10 minutes. Turn each slice then bake for another 5 minutes.

➢ Divide the baked eggplant between each half of the ciabatta roll. Top this with mozzarella, parmesan, and marinara. Place the other half of the ciabatta up top and serve.

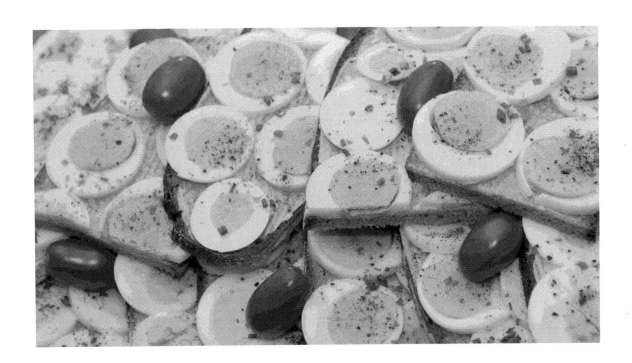

Dinner: Smoked Salmon with Egg Salad (1 point)

Yield: 4 servings

Nutritional Facts: calories: 312, saturated fat: 4g, total fat: 16g, carbs: 8g, sugar: 4g, fiber: 4g, protein: 35g, sodium: 1984mg, cholesterol: 346mg

Ingredients:

- 2 tablespoons coarse salt

- 8 cups water

- 8 eggs

- 1 ½ pound asparagus, cut

- 1 pound smoked salmon

- 2 teaspoons chopped chives

- 2 teaspoons lemon zest

- 1/8 teaspoon ground black pepper

- 2 teaspoons extra virgin olive oil

- ½ lemon's juice

Directions:

➤ Fill a pot with 8 cups of water and boil. After it boils, add the salt and cook the asparagus for 5 minutes. Leave the water boiling when you take out the asparagus.

➤ Drain the asparagus and place it in an ice bath. In the pot of boiling water, cook the eggs for 6 minutes.

➤ Drain the water and allow eggs to cool before shelling.

➢ On a large plate, place your salmon, eggs, asparagus, chives, lemon zest, pepper, lemon juice, and extra olive oil.

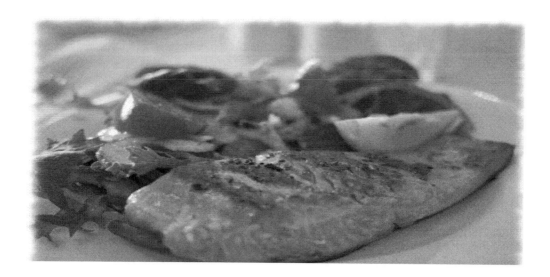

Breakfast: Blueberry Oat Pancakes (12 points)

Yield: 4 servings

Nutritional Facts: calories: 304, saturated fat: 10g, total fat: 14g, trans fat: 0g, sodium: 458mg, cholesterol: 50mg, fiber: 6g, carbs: 36g, protein: 12g, sugar: 13g

Ingredients:

- ½ cup rolled oats

- ½ cup white whole wheat flour

- ¼ cup coconut flour

- 2 teaspoons baking powder

- 1 tablespoon honey

- ½ teaspoon salt

- ½ cup skim milk

- 1 cup plain Greek yogurt

- 1 lightly beaten egg

- 2 tablespoons melted coconut oil

- 1 cup blueberries

Directions:

➤ Combine all of the ingredients in a bowl, except for the blueberries. After everything's mixed, fold in the blueberries.

➤ Use a non-stick spray on a skillet. Pour about ¼ cup of your batter and cook each side is golden.

➤ Serve with fruit toppings, some honey, or maple syrup.

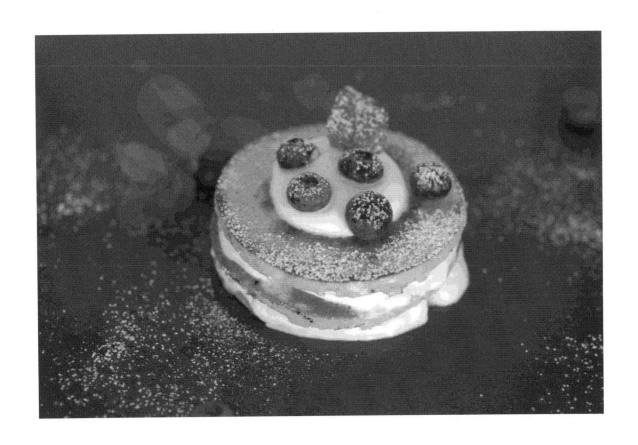

Lunch: Instant Pot Creamy Spaghetti (10 points)

Yield: 8 servings

Nutritional Facts: calories: 348, saturated fat: 1g, total fat: 7g, trans fat: 0g, sugar: 8g, carbs: 51g, protein: 20g, fiber: 4g, sodium: 762mg, cholesterol: 44mg

Ingredients:

- 1 box whole wheat spaghetti pasta

- 1 pound ground turkey sausage

- 1 jar no-sugar marinara sauce

- 1 can diced tomatoes

- 4 cups water

Directions:

➢ Set Instant Pot to sauté mode then add the turkey sausage. Cook then break into small pieces. Drain excess liquid.

➢ Break the spaghetti in half and place this in the Instant Pot. Add water, diced tomatoes, and marinara sauce. Cover pasta in liquid.

➢ Set Instant Pot to manual mode and high pressure. Set timer for 8 minutes. Once done, remove the lid and mix well.

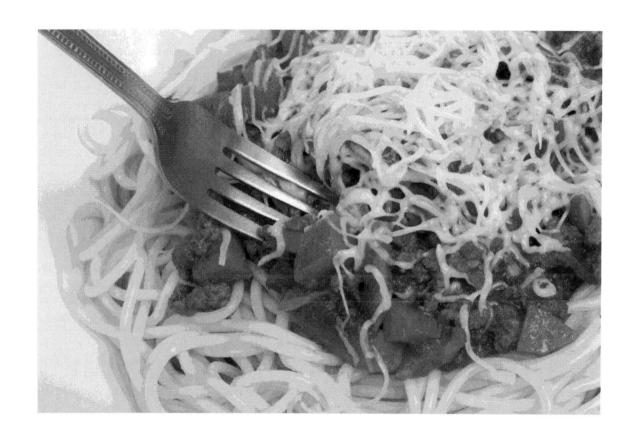

Dinner: Slow Cooker Chicken Enchiladas (9 points)

Yield: 4

Nutritional Facts: calories: 393, saturated fat: 5g, total fat: 11g, trans fat: 0g, fiber: 5g, carbs, 34g, protein: 38g, sugar: 10g, sodium: 1249mg, cholesterol: 104mg

Ingredients:

- 1 cup shredded chicken

- ½ teaspoon ground cumin

- ¼ teaspoon garlic powder

- Salt and black pepper

- 1/3 cup reduced fat cheddar cheese, shredded and divided

- 1 cup sugar-free red enchilada sauce, divided

- ¼ cup Greek yogurt, divided

- Shredded lettuce and diced tomatoes

- 4 small whole grain tortillas

Directions:

➢ Combine the chicken, cumin, garlic powder, salt, and pepper.

➢ Add half the enchilada sauce, half the Greek yogurt, and half the cheddar cheese. Mix well.

➢ Divide this mixture equally for each tortilla. Place it in the center. Roll it up and place in a slow cooker.

➤ Combine the yogurt and enchilada sauce together. Pour this on the enchiladas and cook on low for 3 hours—or until it becomes bubbly.

➤ Plate this after, pouring the liquid from the slow cooker on the enchiladas. Top with cheese, shredded lettuce, and tomatoes.

Breakfast: Dairy Free Crepes (5 points)

Yield: 4

Nutritional Facts: calories 190, saturated fat: 1g, total fat: 7g, trans fat: 0g, fiber: 1g, carbs: 25g, protein: 6g, sugar: 1g

Ingredients:

- 1 ¼ cup water

- 1 cup flour

- 1 ¼ teaspoon sugar

- 2 eggs

- 1 ¼ tablespoons olive oil, divided

- Salt

Directions:

➢ Mix the water, eggs, flour, sugar, salt, and 1 tablespoon of olive oil until it becomes smooth. Keep in the fridge for half an hour.

➢ After half an hour, oil a saucepan or skillet using the remaining olive oil. Get rid of any excess with a paper towel.

➢ Pour a portion of the crepe batter then swirl it on the skillet to distribute evenly. Flip to cook both sides properly.

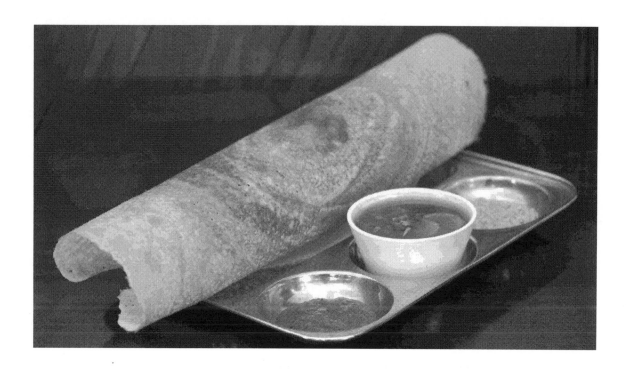

Lunch: Chicken and Spinach Ramen Bowl (5 points)

Yield: 4

Nutritional Facts: calories: 275, saturated fat: 3g, total fat: 11g, trans fat: 0g, carbs: 20g, cholesterol: 52mg, sugar: 2g, fiber: 2g, protein: 25g, sodium: 780mg

Ingredients:

- 2 garlic cloves, minced

- 1 tablespoon fresh ginger, minced

- 2 tablespoons soy sauce

- 4 cups low sodium chicken broth

- 1 teaspoon curry powder

- ¼ cup rice vinegar

- 2 skinless, boneless chicken breast, cut into 1 inch cubes

- Tablespoon sesame oil

- 1 cup sliced fresh mushrooms

- 1 pack ramen noodles, discard seasoning packet

- 3 cups baby spinach

- ¼ cup chopped green onion

- ¼ cup shredded carrot

- 2 tablespoons chopped cilantro

- 1 sliced jalapeno pepper

Directions:

➢ Set Insta Pot to the manual setting. Mix your garlic, ginger, soy sauce, chicken broth, curry powder, vinegar, chicken, sesame oil, and mushrooms together. Set the pressure to high for 10 minutes.

➢ Once done, stir in the ramen noodles and the spinach. Place back the lid and let these sit in the hot broth for 5 minutes.

➢ Top each bowl with green onions, carrots, cilantro, and jalapeno.

Dinner: Creamy Chicken and Mushrooms (2 points)

Yield: 4

Nutritional Facts: calories: 291, saturated fat: 1g, total fat: 6g, fiber: 1g, carbs: 8g, sugar: 5g, fiber: 1g, protein: 48g, sodium: 824mg, cholesterol: 131mg

Ingredients:

- 4 skinless and boneless chicken breast

- 1 ½ cups chicken broth

- 2 cups sliced mushrooms

- 1 teaspoon salt

- ½ teaspoon dried thyme

- ½ teaspoon ground black pepper

- 1 teaspoon garlic powder

- ¼ cup fat free cream cheese

- 2 teaspoons Worcestershire sauce

- ½ cup plain fat free Greek yogurt

Directions:

➢ Place all of the ingredients, except for the yogurt and cream cheese in a slow cooker. Cook on high for 3 hours.

➢ Remove chicken from slow cooker then set aside. Whisk in the yogurt and cream cheese until it becomes smooth. Bring back the chicken and cook for another 15 minutes.

➢ Serve and top with cheese.

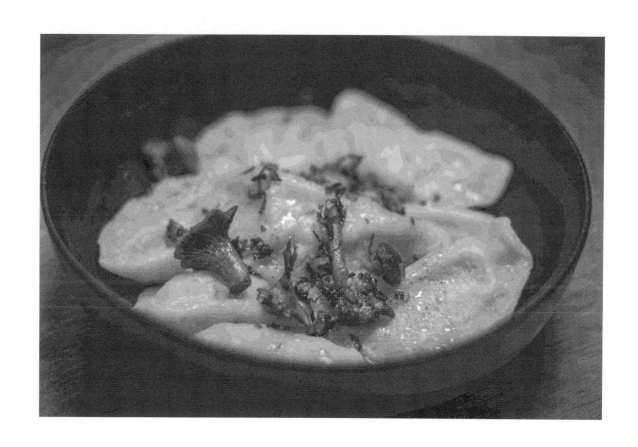

Breakfast: Avocado Stuffed Deviled Eggs (1 points)

Yield: 12

Nutritional Facts: calories 94, saturated fat: 2g, total fat: 7g, trans fat: 0g, fiber: 1g, carbs: 3g, protein: 6g, sugar: 1g, sodium: 151mg, cholesterol: 149mg.

Ingredients:

- ½ a peeled avocado, mashed

- 6 hard-boiled eggs, cut lengthwise in half

- 1 teaspoon Dijon mustard

- ½ teaspoon lemon juice

- ½ teaspoon salt

- 1 clove garlic

- ¼ cup chopped green onion

- 1 teaspoon smoked paprika

Directions:

➢ Remove the yolks from the hardboiled eggs carefully. Place this in a large bowl and the other half on a separate platter.

➢ Add your avocado, Dijon, lemon juice, and garlic to the yolks. Mash this until smooth. Using a piping bag or a spoon, fill the centers of each egg half with the mixture. Dust this with paprika and some green onion. Serve cold.

Lunch: Spinach and Mozzarella Frittata (3 points)

Yield: 6

Nutritional Facts: calories: 139, saturated fat: 1g, total fat: 8g, trans fat: 0g, carbs: 4g, cholesterol: 94mg, sugar: 2g, fiber: 1g, protein: 12g

Ingredients:

- ½ cup diced onion

- 1 tablespoon extra-virgin olive oil

- 3 egg whites

- 3 eggs

- 1 cup shredded mozzarella, divided

- 1 tablespoons milk

- ¼ teaspoon white pepper

- ¼ teaspoon black pepper

- 1 diced roma tomato

- 1 cup baby spinach, chopped

- Salt

Directions:

➢ On a small skillet, add your oil and then sauté the onions until tender.

➢ Using a non-stick spray or olive oil, spray the inside of your slow cooker.

➢ Combine the sautéed onions, the ¾ cup mozzarella cheese, and the rest of your ingredients. Whisk and pour this into the slow cooker. Sprinkle the rest of the cheese on top.

➢ Cook on low for 1 to 1 ½ hours until eggs set.

Dinner: Squash Gnocchi and Sage Butter Sauce (10 points)

Yield: 4

Nutritional Facts: calories: 359, saturated fat: 14g, total fat: 23g, trans fat: 1g, fiber: 7g, carbs: 35g, sugar: 6g, fiber: 7g, protein: 10g, sodium: 773mg, cholesterol: 95mg

Ingredients:

- 2 ½ pounds butternut squash, seeded and sliced

- 1 egg

- 10 ounces floor, plus extra for sprinkling

- 1 ¼ teaspoons salt

- 3 ounces low fat butter

- ¼ teaspoon nutmeg powder

- ½ cup grated romano cheese

- 10 fresh sage leaves

Directions:

➢ Preheat oven to 400 degrees. Place the squash with skin on a baking tray. Bake for 45 minutes to 1 hour, this varies depending on the thickness of the squash.

➢ After, peel skin away and mix the pulp with egg, flour, ¼ teaspoon salt, and nutmeg.

➢ Knead until you have a compact dough. Add more flour if it's still sticky.

➢ Divide this dough into several equal parts. Roll each one to make a cylindrical shape and slice to smaller pieces.

➢ Sprinkle flour on it to keep it from sticking together.

➢ Boil water in a large pot. While waiting, prepare the sauce. In a saucepan, melt butter and heat this with the sage. Keep it warm.

➢ Add gnocchi to the water, sprinkle some salt, and cook for 3 minutes. Remove then transfer to the saucepan, coat evenly.

➢ Serve and top with cheese.

Breakfast: Peach Pie Breakfast Parfait (10 points)

Yield: 4

Nutritional Facts: calories: 260, saturated fat: 4g, total fat: 13g, trans fat: 0g, sodium: 20mg, cholesterol: 0mg, fiber: 8g, carbs: 30g, protein: 6g, sugar: 13g

Ingredients:

- ¼ cup chia seeds

- 1 cup coconut milk

- 1 tablespoon pure maple syrup

- 1 teaspoon ground cinnamon

- 2/3 cup granola

- 1 diced medium peaches

Directions:

➢ Combine the chia seeds, coconut milk, and maple syrup. Cover this and keep in the fridge for an hour.

➢ Toss cinnamon and peaches together. Set aside as well.

➢ Divide the milk and chia mixture between two containers. Top this with granola, but set aside 2 tablespoons of it. Divide the peaches equally between containers and top with the rest of the granola.

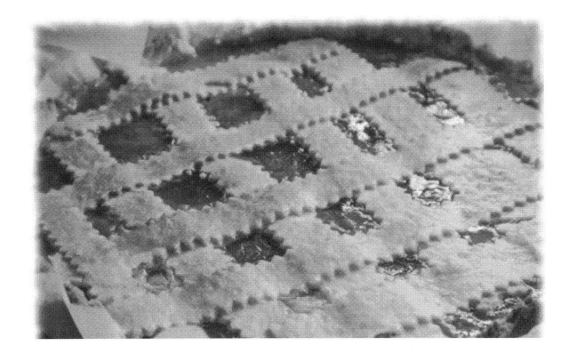

Lunch: French Onion Soup Casserole (7 points)

Yield: 4

Nutritional Facts: calories: 275, saturated fat: 4g, total fat: 13g, trans fat: 0g, fiber: 3g, carbs: 28g, protein: 13g, sugar: 8g, sodium: 796mg, cholesterol: 19mg

Ingredients:

- 3 large onions, sliced thinly

- 2 tablespoons olive oil

- 4 cups low sodium beef broth (vegetable can be used too)

- 1 teaspoon dried thyme leaves

- 1 teaspoon Worcestershire sauce

- 10 slices of whole wheat baguette

- ¼ cup chopped parsley leaves

- ¾ cup low fat shredded mozzarella

Directions:

➢ Preheat oven to 400 degrees.

➢ Prepare a large skillet. Put olive oil on it and set to medium heat. Add the onions and cook for 30 minutes until soft. Add the Worcestershire, broth, and thyme leaves. Allow to boil.

➢ Place baguettes on baking sheet and bake until crisp. Pour onion mix onto the baguette and sprinkle mozzarella on top. Bake for another 30 minutes until cheese is bubbly.

➢ Top with parsley and thyme.

Dinner: BBQ Chicken and Avocado Quesadillas (9 points)

Yield: 6

Nutritional Facts: calories: 271, saturated fat: 5g, total fat: 14g, trans fat: 0g, sodium: 414mg, cholesterol: 41mg, fiber: 4g, carbs: 24g, protein: 14g, sugar: 9g

<u>Ingredients:</u>

- 1 large chicken breast with skin

- 1 diced avocado

- ½ cup barbecue sauce

- 6 whole grain tortillas

- 1 cup shredded mozzarella

Directions:

➤ Preheat oven to 375 degrees

➤ Add chicken breast and ¼ cup water to a casserole plan. Loosely cover with foil and bake for 45 minutes. Let chicken cool before shredding it with fork. Discard skin.

➤ Combine shredded chicken with barbecue sauce.

➤ Heat tortillas. On one half, sprinkle a tablespoon of mozzarella, 1/6th of the diced avocado, 1/6th of the chicken mixture, then top with cheese before folding tortilla.

➤ Cook both sides evenly until golden and cheese is melted.

Breakfast: Gingerbread Pancakes (3 points)

Yield: 4

Nutritional Facts: calories: 164, total fat: 3.1g, cholesterol: 0g, carbs: 26.9g, sodium: 146mg, sugar: 6.6g, dietary fiber: 7.0g, protein: 8.7g

Ingredients:

- 2/3 cup unsweetened almond milk

- 1 tablespoon blackstrap molasses

- ¼ cup egg whites

- 1 tablespoon chia seed

- 10 drops vanilla stevia

- 1 teaspoon gluten-free pure vanilla extract

- 1 teaspoon gluten-free baking powder

- 2/3 cup chickpea flour

- 1 teaspoon ground ginger

- 1 teaspoon ground cinnamon

- 1/8 teaspoon ground cloves

Directions:

➢ Combine chia and milk. Let sit for 10 minutes. You can also soak the chia overnight in the milk.

➢ Preheat non-stick pan on low for 2 minutes.

➢ Combine all the dry ingredients in one bowl. Transfer to wet ingredients after.

➤ Mix well then pour ¼ of the mixture onto the pan. Cook sides evenly until bubbles form and edges turn golden.

➤ Serve topped with apples, pecans, maple syrup, and coconut oil. Optional.

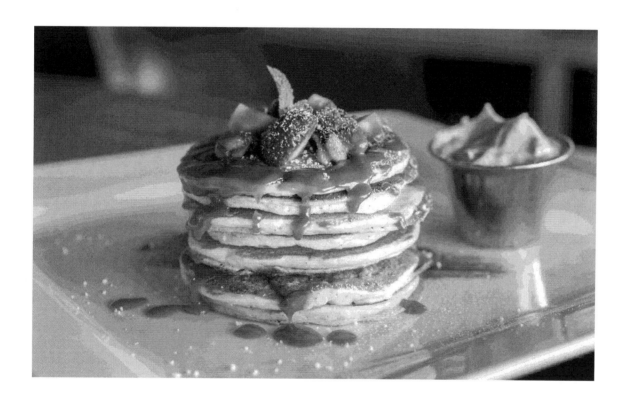

Lunch: Pita Pocket Breakfast Sandwich (6 points)

Yield: 2

Nutritional Facts: calories: 297, total fat: 12g, cholesterol: 225mg, carbs: 21g, sodium: 484mg, sugar: 2g, dietary fiber: 3g, protein: 21g

Ingredients:

- 2 large egg whites

- 2 large eggs

- 1 tablespoon milk

- 4 cherry tomatoes sliced in half

- 1 cup torn baby spinach

- Salt and pepper

- 2 diced green onions

- ¼ cup feta cheese crumbles

- 2 teaspoons olive oil

- 1 whole wheat pita pocket, halved

Directions:

➤ Preheat oven to 350 degrees.

➤ Whisk eggs, egg whites, spinach, milk, green onions, tomatoes, salt, and pepper. Pour mixture on a skillet and place in the oven. Leave enough space for the pita bread on the rack.

➤ Brush olive oil on either half of the pita and place in foil. Warm these in the oven during the final 2 minutes of cooking. Sprinkle feta cheese then place back in the oven for another minute.

➤ Cut omelet in half and place one in each pita pocket. Serve hot.

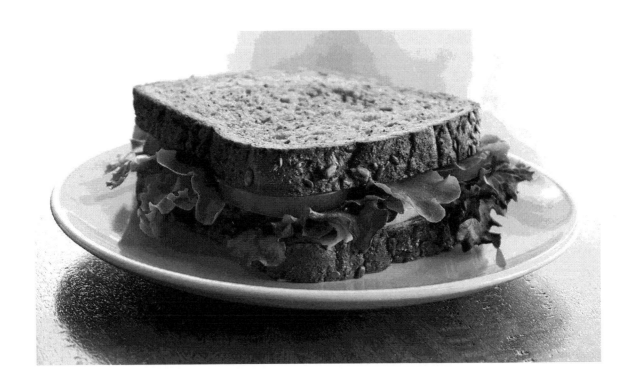

Dinner: Southwest Veggie Wraps (6 points)

Yield: 4

Nutritional Facts: calories: 369, carbs: 60g, total fat: 8g, sugar: 5g, fiber: 11g, sodium: 439mg, protein: 16g

Ingredients:

- 1 tablespoon olive oil

- 1 green bell pepper, sliced thinly

- 1 red onion, sliced thinly

- 1 cup black beans

- ½ cup carrot, shredded

- 1 cup cooked black beans

- 1 tablespoon chili powder

- 1 teaspoon ground cumin

- ½ teaspoon salt

- 1 jalapeno pepper

- 2 cup chopped kale

- ¼ cup fresh cilantro

- 4 whole wheat flour tortillas

Directions:

➤ Heat olive oil on medium heat. Add bell pepper, onion, and carrot. Cook for 4 minutes then add black beans, chili powder, cumin, jalapeno, kale, and salt. Cook for another 5 minutes.

➤ Stir in cilantro.

➢ Arrange the tortillas and divide the veggie mix evenly between each one. Fold the sides after and roll into a burrito shape.

Breakfast: Ham and Poached Egg Muffin (6 points)

Yield: 4

Nutritional Facts: calories: 209, cholesterol: 176mg, total fat: 11g, carbs: 16g, sodium: 503mg, protein: 13g, sugar: 4g, fiber: 3g

Ingredients:

- 1 tomato, cut into 4 thick slices

- 3 teaspoons olive oil

- 2 whole wheat English muffins, cut in halves

- 4 slices low-sodium ham

- ¼ teaspoon ground black pepper

- 4 poached eggs

Directions:

➤ Heat 2 teaspoons of olive oil. Add ham and tomatoes, cook until ham turns golden brown.

➤ Place cooked ham on the English muffin and top with the tomato.

➤ Add poached egg on top and drizzle with olive oil. Sprinkle pepper.

Lunch: Instant Pot Macaroni and Cheese (13 points)

Yield: 8

Nutritional Facts: calories: 396, cholesterol: 91mg, total fat: 17g, sodium: 415mg, fiber: 2g, carbs: 42g, protein: 19g, sugar: 2g

Ingredients:

- 1 box whole wheat macaroni noodles

- 4 cups water

- ½ cup skim milk

- ½ teaspoon salt

- 3 cups fat-free shredded cheddar

- ½ teaspoon ground mustard

Directions:

➢ Mix the water and macaroni in the Instant pot. Set it to manual with high pressure and cook for 5 minutes.

➢ After, remove the lid and stir in the remaining ingredients. Stir properly until cheese melts. If there's too much water in the pot, drain any excess before doing this step.

➢ Serve hot and top with some pepper according to taste.

Dinner: Bean and Potato Soup (8 points)

Yield: 8

Nutritional Facts: calories: 287, cholesterol: 2mg, total fat: 3g, sodium: 92mg, fiber: 10g, carbs: 53g, protein: 13g, sugar: 2g

Ingredients:

- 2 cans northern beans, rinsed and drained

- 1 pound Yukon gold potatoes, peeled and chopped

- ½ cup chopped shallots or onions

- ½ cup chopped carrots

- 2 minced garlic cloves

- ½ cup chopped celery

- 2 tablespoons chopped rosemary or 2 teaspoons dried rosemary

- 2 tablespoons fresh thyme

- ½ tablespoon chopped fresh oregano

- 1 teaspoon sea salt and 1 teaspoon black pepper

- 4 cups low sodium vegetable stock

- 1 teaspoon crushed red pepper flakes (adjust to preference)

- 1 tablespoon extra-virgin olive oil

- 1 piece parmesan

- 1 bay leaf

Directions:

➢ Add all of the ingredients to the crockpot. Mix well and allow to cook on low for 6 hours.

➢ If you want a more savory flavor, add the parmesan rind. Adjust according to taste. Do remove before serving

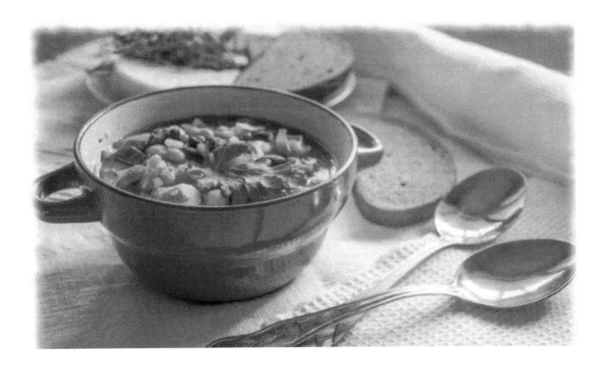

Breakfast: Sweet Potato Breakfast Hash (6 points)

Yield: 6

Nutritional Facts: calories: 186, carbs: 14g, total fat: 11g, fiber: 4g, sodium: 457mg, cholesterol: 22mg, protein: 8g, sugar: 2g

Ingredients:

- 2 large sweet potatoes, peeled and diced

- ½ teaspoon kosher salt

- 3 tablespoons olive oil

- 1 tablespoon apple cider vinegar

- ¼ teaspoon ground white pepper

- 1 teaspoon honey

- 2 minced garlic cloves

- ¼ cup yellow onion, diced

- 8 ounces diced low sodium, sulfate free ham

- ¼ cup green bell pepper, diced

- 1 avocado, diced

- 1 tablespoon lemon juice

Directions:

➢ Preheat oven to 450 degrees.

➢ Coat the sweet potatoes with salt, pepper, and ½ tablespoon of olive oil. Spread evenly on a baking sheet and bake for 15 minutes until potatoes are tender.

➢ Mix the garlic, apple cider vinegar, and honey. Whisk while adding 1 tablespoon of olive oil. Set aside.

➢ On a skillet, heat the rest of the olive oil. Add the green pepper and onion. Cook until onions are soft then add the ham. Remove from heat then stir the apple cider vinegar sauce.

➢ Combine avocado and lemon juice. Stir into the hash.

Lunch: Instant Pot Jambalaya (7 points)

Yield: 6

Nutritional Facts: calories: 399, cholesterol: 167mg, total fat: 7g, sodium: 395mg, fiber: 6g, carbs: 48g, protein: 35g, sugar: 7g

Ingredients:

- 1 tablespoon olive oil

- 2 skinless and boneless chicken breast, cut into cubes

- 1 cup smoked rope sausage, cut into half-moons (preferably low sodium)

- ½ cup chopped red bell pepper

- 1 cup chopped onion

- ½ cup chopped green bell pepper

- 3 minced garlic cloves

- 1 cup chopped celery

- 1 tablespoon Cajun seasoning

- 1 teaspoon dried thyme

- 2 cans low sodium diced tomatoes

- 1 ½ cups brown rice

- 1 cup chicken broth

- 1 teaspoon Worcestershire sauce

- 1 pound raw shrimp, deveined and peeled

- ¼ cup chopped fresh parsley

Directions:

➢ Set Instant Pot to sauté. Ad 1/3 of the oil to the pot then add the sausages. Cook for 5 minutes. Remove sausages then set aside.

➢ Add another 1/3 of the oil to the pot and add the chicken. Cook until it begins to brown. Remove the chicken then set aside.

➢ Heat what remains of the olive oil then toss in the red and green bell peppers, the onion, garlic, and celery. Cook until onions are soft.

➢ Stir in the Cajun seasoning, thyme, and rice. Mix until everything is evenly coated. Add the cooked chicken and sausage. Toss in the rest of the ingredients save for the parsley.

➤ Change setting to manual with high pressure and leave for 7 minutes.

➤ Serve hot and top with fresh parsley.

Dinner: Crispy Zucchini Tacos (8 points)

Yield: 6

Nutritional Facts: calories: 286, cholesterol: 3mg, total fat: 10g, sodium: 240mg, protein: 9g, carbs: 44g, sugar: 3g, fiber: 6g

Ingredients:

(Zucchini)

- 1 cup whole wheat panko bread crumbs

- 3 egg whites

- ¼ cup whole wheat flour

- 1 teaspoon ground cumin

- 2 teaspoons chili powder

- ¼ teaspoon salt

- 1 large zucchini squash, cut into long strips

- ¼ teaspoon pepper

- 3 tablespoons melted coconut oil

(Chipotle Cream)

- ½ cup plain Greek yogurt

- 1 teaspoon lime juice

- 2 tablespoons pureed chipotle peppers

(Tacos)

- 1 cup red cabbage

- 12 corn tortillas

- ½ cup halved cherry tomatoes

- ½ cup sliced radish

- ½ cup chopped fresh cilantro

- 2 tablespoons lemon juice

Directions:

(Zucchini)

➤ Preheat oven to 400 degrees.

➤ Whip egg whites then set aside. In a separate bowl, combine flour, chili powder, panko, salt, pepper, and cumin.

➤ Dip the zucchini pieces in the egg, followed by the flour mixture. Make sure all sides are coated well.

➤ Spread this on a baking sheet then drizzle with coconut oil. Bake until golden brown.

(Chipotle Cream)

➢ Whisk all the ingredients well and set aside.

(Tacos)

➢ Add a cooked zucchini on each tortilla. Top this with radish, tomato, cabbage, and cilantro. Drizzle with chipotle cream and lime juice.

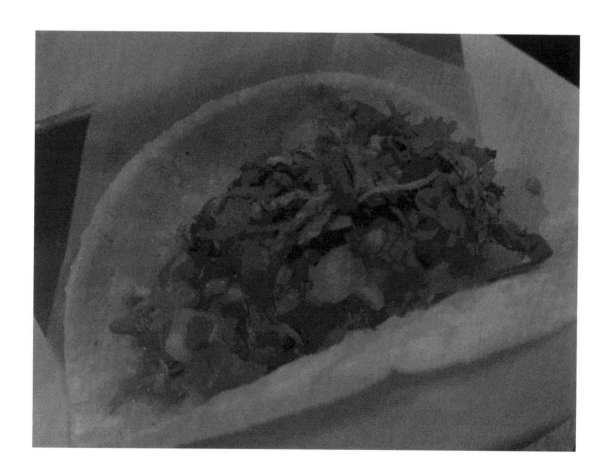

Breakfast: Baked Peanut Butter Banana Oatmeal (11 points)

Yield: 8

Nutritional Facts: calories: 295, cholesterol: 20mg, total fat: 15g, sodium: 76mg, fiber: 5g, carbs: 35g, protein: 9g, sugar: 11g

Ingredients:

- 1 cup oats

- ¾ cup almond milk

- 1/3 cup coconut sugar

- 1 egg

- 2 tablespoons melted coconut oil

- 1 teaspoon baking powder

- ½ cup no-sugar peanut butter

- 1 teaspoon vanilla

- 1 sliced medium banana

Directions:

➢ Heat oven to 350 degrees. Prepare a baking pan with non-stick spray.

➢ Combine all the ingredients save for the banana. Spread it in an even layer on the baking pan. Layer sliced bananas on top then bake for 20 minutes.

➢ Let sit for 10 minutes before cutting and serving.

Lunch: Black Bean and Sweet Potato Wrap (13 points)

Yield: 4

Nutritional Facts: calories: 396, cholesterol: 1mg, total fat: 14g, carbs: 58g, sodium: 155mg, sugar: 5g, fiber: 9g, protein: 11g

Ingredients:

- 1 tablespoon coconut oil

- ½ cup chopped sweet potatoes

- ½ cup drained black beans

- Juice of 1 lime

- 1 teaspoon taco seasoning

- ½ diced avocado

- ½ cup diced tomatoes

- ¼ cup diced red onion

- 2 whole grain wraps

- 3 tablespoons fat free Greek yogurt

- Salt and pepper

Directions:

➢ Stir Greek yogurt, lime juice, and taco seasoning together. Keep in the fridge until ready to use.

➢ Heat oil in a skillet. Toss sweet potatoes in and cook until tender and slightly browned. Salt and pepper as preferred.

➤ Toss together sweet potatoes and black beans in a separate bowl. Drizzle remaining lime juice. Salt and pepper, if needed.

➤ Spread Greek yogurt on each wrap. Top this with sweet potato mixture, onions, avocado, and tomatoes. Roll and cut in half before serving.

Dinner: Caprese Pasta (12 points)

Yield: 6

Nutritional Facts: calories: 392, cholesterol: 30mg, total fat: 10g, carbs: 57g, sodium: 571mg, protein: 18g, fiber: 3g, sugar: 5g

Ingredients:

- 1 pound whole grain spaghetti

- 2 cups chopped basil (keep extra for garnish)

- 3 cups cherry tomatoes, sliced

- 1 teaspoon salt, ½ teaspoon pepper

- 3 minced garlic cloves

- 8 ounces shredded mozzarella

- 1 tablespoon balsamic vinegar

Directions:

➤ Put the spaghetti, water, tomatoes, garlic, basil, red pepper flakes, salt, and pepper into a pot. Let this boil then continue cooking for 13 minutes until the pasta is thoroughly cooked.

➤ Drain excess water and top with balsamic vinegar, mozzarella, and garnish with basil.

➤ Let cheese melt before serving.

Breakfast: Three Seed Berry Parfait (6 points)

Yield: 6

Nutritional Facts: calories: 128, cholesterol: 5mg, total fat: 3g, carbs: 21g, sodium: 59mg, fiber: 3g, protein: 6g, sugar: 17g

Ingredients:

- 2 tablespoons honey

- 2 cups fat free Greek yogurt

- 1 cup blueberries

- 1 cup raspberries

- 1 cup sliced strawberries

- 1 tablespoon chia seeds

- 1 tablespoon ground flax seeds

- 1 tablespoon hemp seeds

- 2 tablespoons lemon juice

Directions:

➢ Mix the lemon juice, honey, and yogurt. Stir well

➢ Layer the berries, seeds, and yogurt mix in a parfait glass. Sprinkle seeds on top.

Lunch: Mediterranean Quinoa Bowl (5 points)

Yield: 6

Nutritional Facts: calories: 181, cholesterol: 0mg, total fat: 8g, carbs: 23g, sugar: 1g, fiber: 5g, protein: 6g, sodium: 225mg

Ingredients:

- ½ small onion

- 2 tablespoons olive oil

- 2 cups baby spinach

- 1 minced garlic clove

- ½ pitted Kalamata olives

- ½ cup drained artichoke hearts

- Juice of 1 lemon

- 1 cup cooked white beans

- Salt and pepper

Directions:

➢ Over medium heat, prepare a skillet with olive oil. Cook the onions on it until soft then add the garlic. Cook for another minute then add the spinach.

➢ When the spinach wilts, stir in the quinoa and cook for 2 minutes. Add the olives, artichokes, and white beans. Season this with pepper and drizzle lemon juice before serving.

Dinner: Shrimp Stir-Fry (1 points)

Yield: 5 cups

Nutritional Facts: calories: 117, cholesterol: 103mg, total fat: 2gm, sodium: 272mg, fiber: 1mg, carbs: 10mg, protein: 15mg, sugar: 6mg

Ingredients:

- 2 tablespoons water

- 2 tablespoons cornstarch

- 2 hoisin sauce

- 2 tablespoons soy sauce

- ¼ cup low sodium chicken broth

- 1 teaspoons sesame oil

- 1 tablespoon minced ginger

- 4 thinly sliced green onions

- 1 ½ uncooked shrimp

- ½ pound fresh snow peas

- 2 minced garlic cloves

- Toasted sesame seeds

- 1 tablespoon minced fresh ginger

- Serve over brown rice noodles, brown rice, or soba

Directions:

Combine sesame oil, honey, hoisin sauce, soy sauce, water, and cornstarch in a bowl. Whisk until smooth.

Stir fry shrimp in 1 teaspoon sesame oil with chicken broth. Cook for 3 minutes until shrimp turns pink. Remove and set aside.

➢ Add green onion to the skillet and fry for 3 minutes. Add snow peas and stir until peas are tender. Add ginger root and garlic. Cook for another 2 minutes.

➢ Add sauce mixture to the skillet and simmer. Add shrimp and heat.

➢ Place over brown rice and top with sesame seeds.

Breakfast: Honey Nut Breakfast Cereal (8 points)

Yield: 12

Nutritional Facts: calories: 202, cholesterol: 0mg, total fat: 10g, carbs: 27g, sodium: 1mg, protein: 4g, fiber: 3g, sugar: 8g

Ingredients:

- ¼ cup raw walnuts

- 4 cups old fashioned oats

- ¼ cup raw almonds

- 1/3 cup raw honey

- 1 teaspoon cinnamon

- 1/3 cup melted coconut oil

Directions:

➢ Preheat oven to 325 degrees

➢ Mix dry ingredients and stir well. Add coconut oil and honey together, mix thoroughly with the oats until it is evenly covered. Make sure the oats are moist.

➢ Spread the cereal mixture on a lined cookie sheet. Bake this and stir every 10 minutes until it becomes golden brown. This should take around 30 minutes.

➢ Store these in an airtight container. You can include dried fruit or raisins before adding low fat milk.

➢ If you're not keen on nuts, you can switch it to ¼ cup of raw sunflower seeds, ¼ cup sesame seeds, and ¼ cup raw pumpkin seeds. You can also use ¼ cup edamame instead of nuts. These would provide similar nutritional value and protein.

Lunch: Savory Mexican Oats (2 points)

Yield: 4

Nutritional Facts: calories: 159, cholesterol: 0mg, total fat: 3g, carbs: 29g, sodium: 507mg, fiber: 5g, protein: 8g, sugar: 5g

Ingredients:

- 1 cup salsa

- 1 cup steel cut oats

- 2 cups low sodium chicken broth

- 2 tablespoons chopped cilantro

- 1 cup chopped red pepper

- 1 cup thawed frozen corn

Directions:

➤ Mix all the ingredients together and place in your slow cooker.

➤ Set the timer for 2 to 4 hours or however long it takes for the oats to completely cook

➤ Set the temperature to low

Dinner: Baked Chicken and Vegetable Spring Rolls (3 points)

Yield: 8

Nutritional Facts: calories: 127, cholesterol: 11mg, fiber: 1g, protein: 4g, sugar: 2g, sodium: 368mg

Ingredients:

- 1 finely chopped garlic clove

- 3 tablespoons extra virgin olive oil

- 1 finely chopped onion

- 1 cup julienned carrots

- 4 ounces diced chicken fillet

- 1 cup julienne cabbage

- 1 cup string beans

- ¼ teaspoon salt

- 3 tablespoons soy sauce

- ¼ teaspoon ground pepper

- 8 spring roll wrappers

Directions:

➢ Preheat oven to 400 degrees

➢ In a large saucepan, heat extra virgin olive oil then sauté the onion and garlic for a minute

➢ Add the chicken and cook for another 5 minutes

➢ Add the rest of the veggies and continue sautéing for 15 minutes

➤ Add the soy sauce, pepper, and salt. Toss for 1 minute then set aside.

➤ Begin making the rolls. Make sure that the chicken mixture has cooled down a bit before you begin working on this.

➤ Line a baking tray with parchment and place the spring rolls on it

➤ Brush each roll with extra virgin olive oil

➤ Bake for 15 to 20 minutes until the rolls become golden brown

➤ Serve this with your desired dipping sauce

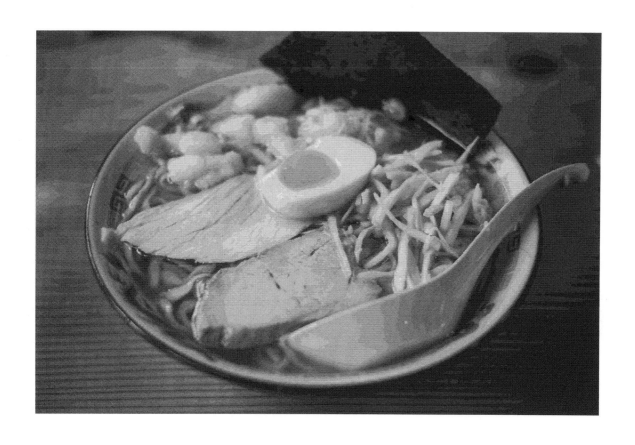

Breakfast: Crustless Vegetable Quiche (2 points)

Yield: 6

Nutritional Facts: calories: 141, cholesterol: 93mg, carbohydrates: 15g, sodium: 593mg, fiber: 5, protein: 11g, sugar: 5g

Ingredients:

- 1 small diced yellow onion

- 1 tablespoon olive oil

- 1 minced garlic clove

- ½ cup zucchini

- ½ cup diced green bell pepper

- ½ cup diced red bell pepper

- ¼ cup diced sun-dried tomatoes

- 6 broccoli florets

- 4 large egg whites

- 3 large eggs

- 1 teaspoon oregano

- 2 tablespoons low fat milk

- Salt and ½ teaspoon black pepper

- ¼ cup low fat parmesan cheese

Directions:

➤ Preheat oven to 425 degrees.

➤ Take a large skillet and add oil to it. Sauté garlic and onion until tender. Add zucchini, bell pepper, sun-dried tomatoes, and broccoli. Continue to sauté for another 2 minutes.

➤ Whisk eggs, egg whites, spices, milk, and ¼ cup parmesan cheese together. In a pie dish, add the sautéed vegetables and pour the egg mixture on top of it. Make sure it is covered evenly.

➤ Loosely cover this while foil then bake for around 10 minutes at 425 degrees. Reduce the heat after and lower it to 350. Continue baking this for another 20 to 25 minutes. Remove the foil during the last few minutes of baking, then sprinkle what remains of the cheese on top.

➤ Note that the quiche is done with it puffs up.

Lunch: White Chicken Enchiladas (12 points)

Yield: 8

Nutritional Facts: calories: 316, cholesterol: 62mg, total fat: 17g, carbs: 24g, sodium: 380mg, protein: 18g, fiber: 2g, sugar: 11g

Ingredients:

- 1 teaspoon divided cumin

- 2 cups shredded chicken breast

- 1 teaspoon chili powder

- 1 ½ cups shredded Mexican style cheese

- ½ cup salsa

- 2 tablespoons flour

- 2 tablespoons butter

- 2 cups chicken broth

- 1 container sour cream

- 1 can diced green chilies

- ½ teaspoon black pepper

- ½ teaspoon sea salt

- ¼ cup chopped cilantro

- 8 whole grain tortillas

Directions:

➢ Preheat oven to 375 degrees. Next, combine the chicken with salsa, cumin, and chili powder. Spread the mixture over the tortillas, roll it up, and place in a casserole pan.

➢ Melt butter over medium low heat and sprinkle in the flour. Cook this for 1 minute while stirring. Pour in the chicken broth and stir until it thickens. Add another half teaspoon of cumin, green chilies, 1 cup cheese, salt, pepper, and sour cream.

➢ Pour the white sauce over enchiladas and sprinkle ½ cup of cheese on top. Bake this for 25 minutes until the cheese is golden. Sprinkle cilantro up top.

Dinner: Chicken and Broccoli Stir Fry (8 points)

Yield: 4

Nutritional Facts: calories: 256, cholesterol: 32mg, total fat: 18mg, sodium: 475mg, fiber: 1g, carbs: 15g, protein: 11g, sugar: 6g

Ingredients:

- 2 teaspoon sesame seeds

- 1 tablespoon honey

- 3 tablespoons light soy sauce

- 2 tablespoons sesame oil

- 2 teaspoons lemon

- 1 tablespoon extra-virgin olive oil

- 1 tablespoon cornstarch

- 1 medium coarsely chopped onion

- 1.25 pounds chicken breast filets, chopped

- 1 finely chopped ginger root

- ¼ teaspoon black pepper

- 2 cups broccoli florets

Directions:

➢ Whisk the lemon juice, soy sauce, honey, cornstarch, and sesame oil. Set this aside.

➢ Set a skillet on low heat and toast the sesame seeds for 2 minutes until it becomes fragrant. Place these in a bowl and set aside, too.

➤ To the same skillet, add some olive oil. Turn it to medium heat and cook chicken until it's golden. Add the ginger, pepper, onions, and broccoli. Sauté this for 4 minutes.

➤ Reduce the heat then add your soy sauce, toss then combine. Cook this until the sauce thickens. Make sure that it doesn't exceed 5 minutes. Sprinkle with toasted sesame seeds before serving.

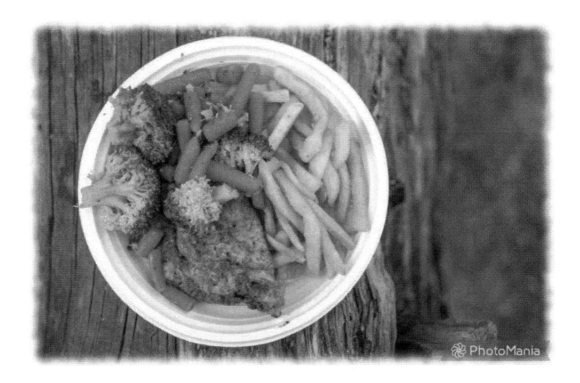

CHAPTER 4

30-day Meal Plan

Using some the recipes provided above, let's move on to creating a sustainable 30-day meal plan which is meant to help you lose weight. Remember, you can always tweak the recipes according to your preference or opt for a different dish depending on the availability of the ingredients.

Note that the other recipes mention on this meal plan can be found on the official Weight Watchers website if you are interested. Should you decide to tweak them, do make sure you opt for the healthier alternative for ingredients as this will affect the overall SmartPoint equivalent of the recipe.

Week 1:

	Sunday	Monday	Tuesday	Wednesday	Thursday	Friday	Saturday
Breakfast	Egg and Spinach Bowl (4pts)	Eggs and Avocado Toast (4pts)	Hot Chocolate Oatmeal (6pts)	Berries, Granola, and Yogurt (5pts)Soufflé Omelet with Mushrooms (1pt)	Cereals and Milk (4pts or less) Reference	Blueberry Oat Pancakes (12pts)	
Lunch	Plant Based Borscht (2pts)	Cheese Pizza (7pts per slice)	Taco Lettuce Boats (3pts)	Grilled Cheese Sandwich (6pts)	Eggplant Parmesan Sandwich (8pts)	Cauliflower Fried Rice (1pt)	Instant Pot Creamy Spaghetti (10pts)
Dinner	Broccoli and Beef Stir Fry (7pts)	Chicken with Mashed Potatoes and Gravy (2pts)	Roast Beef with Side Salad (11pts)	Healthy 4-Ingredient Pesto Pasta (9pts)	Smoked Salmon with Egg Salad (1pt)	WW Pepper Steak (5pts)	Slow Cooker Chicken Enchiladas (9pts)
Total Points	13 points	13 points	20 points	20 points	10 points	10 points	31 points

Note: The points pertain to every single serving that you consume of the meal. So, if you go back for seconds,

148

always multiply the points by two. Of course, these recipes and meal samples were specifically curated to be healthy and help you progress with your weight loss. Just be mindful of your portions and always enjoy your food in moderation.

Week 2:

	Sunday	Monday	Tuesday	Wednesday	Thursday	Friday	Saturday
Breakfast	Peanut Butter and Jelly Sandwich (1pt)	Dairy Free Crepes (5pts)	Cottage Cheese Pancakes (7pts)	Avocado Stuffed Deviled Eggs (1pt)	Pumpkin Spice Waffles (5pts)	Peach Pie Breakfast Parfait (10pts)	Chocolate Banana Smoothie (6pts)
Lunch	Yakisoba Stir Fried Noodles (5pts)	Chicken and Spinach Ramen Bowl (5pts)	Potato Fans with Optional Bacon Bits (6pts)	Spinach and Mozzarella Frittata (3pts)	Grilled Eggplant and Feta Snacks (1pt)	French Onion Soup Casserole (7pts)	Aglio Oglio Spaghetti (2pts)
Dinner	Penne with Peppers and Sausage (6pts)	Creamy Chicken and Mushrooms (2pts)	Grilled Chicken Strips with Salad (6pts)	Squash Gnocchi and Sage Butter Sauce (10pts)	Grilled Salmon with Teriyaki Sauce (4pts)	BBQ Chicken and Avocado Quesadillas (9pts)	Vietnamese Shrimp Spring Rolls (2pts)
Total Points	12 points	12 points	19 points	14 points	10 points	26 points	10 points

Week 3:

	Sunday	Monday	Tuesday	Wednesday	Thursday	Friday	Saturday
Breakfast	Gingerbread Pancakes (3pts)	Bacon and Eggs (2pts)	Ham and Poached Egg Muffin (6 points)	Cinnamon Rolls with Cream Cheese (4pts)	Sweet Potato Breakfast Hash (6 points)	Thyme and Scallion Pancakes (1pt)	Baked Peanut Butter Banana Oatmeal (11 points)
Lunch	Pita Pocket Breakfast Sandwich (6 points)	Mustard Chicken (2pts)	Instant Pot Macaroni and Cheese (13 points)	Bacon Wrapped Pickle Spears (1pt)	Instant Pot Jambalaya (7 points)	Tofu and Vegetable Stir Fry (4pts)	Black Bean and Sweet Potato Wrap (13 points)
Dinner	Southwest Veggie Wraps (6 points)	Shrimp Pad Thai (9pts)	Bean and Potato Soup (8 points)	Slow Cooker Ravioli with Tomato Sauce (9pts)	Crispy Zucchini Tacos (8 points)	Pasta with Clams in White Wine Sauce (9pts)	Caprese Pasta (12 points)
Total Points	15 points	13 points	27 points	14 points	21 points	14 points	36 points

Week 4:

	Sunday	Monday	Tuesday	Wednesday	Thursday	Friday	Saturday
Breakfast	Three Seed Berry Parfait (6 points)	Bacon and Eggs (2pts)	Honey Nut Breakfast Cereal (8 pts)	Greek Yogurt Pancakes (1pt)	Turkey Sausage and Cheddar Omelet (2 pts)	Baked Chocolate Donuts (3pt)	Warm Bacon Breakfast Salad (4pts)
Lunch	Mediterranean Quinoa Bowl (5 points)	Mustard Chicken (2pts)	Savory Mexican Oats (2 pts)	Sheet Pan Chicken Parmesan (5pts)	Garlic Parm Shrimp 4 points)	Cilantro Lime Chicken Kabobs (2pts)	Slow Cooker Turkey Tacos (5 points)
Dinner	Shrimp Stir-Fry (1 points)	Shrimp Pad Thai (9pts)	Baked Chicken and Vegetable Spring Rolls (3 pts)	Turkey Chili (1pt)	Herb, Tomato, and Goat Cheese Frittata (3 pts)	Slow Cooker Black Beans (0pts)	Ground Turkey and Butternut Squash Skillet (3 pts)
Total Points	12 points	13 points	12 points	7 points	9 points	5 points	12 points

For the final two days of this meal plan, we have also included options for desserts and snacks. Use this as a template for what you can add to the other 28 days, should you feel the need for something extra. Remember, it's all about choosing healthy options and making sure that you don't overindulge.

	Sunday	Monday
Breakfast	Go-Lean Fruit and Yogurt Parfait (3pts)	Egg, Cheese, and Veggie Roll-Up (4pts)
Lunch	Garlic Cheese and Bacon Stuffed Chicken Breast (4pts)	Chicken Philly Style Stuffed Peppers (3pts)
Dinner	Buffalo Chicken Rolls (4pts)	Monte Cristo Flatout Sandwich (4pts)
Snack	Easy Pizza Twists (2pts)	Apple Cinnamon French Toast Sandwich (4pts)
Total Points	13 points	15 points

CHAPTER 5

Grocery Buying Guide

Let's talk groceries and stocking up your pantry. At first, this would feel a little challenging. Sure, there are no restrictions when it comes to what you can and cannot eat—but since you're going the healthy route, there are things you would want to stay away from.

- Say NO to canned meat as much as you can. We all know that many of these canned goods contain stuff (preservatives) that's bad for us. Not to mention the fact that they tend to have high sodium content.

- Always have GREENS on hand. They may not keep very long, but these are among the most versatile food items you can have. Toss them in a salad, add them to your burgers, your stews, your rice bowls—the possibilities are endless. They tie with eggs and potatoes when it comes to versatility.

- Want a healthy snack? Try mixed nuts. Get these at your local bulk store, they're usually more affordable there. Pack some up and take it with you to work, to the gym, during your trips, or simply have some at home when you're craving. These can be cooked, dressed, and prepared in many different ways—so you can enjoy them without getting bored.

- What's the best oil for cooking? Have some of these handy:

o Nut Oils

o Truffle Oil

o Extra Virgin Olive Oil

o Avocado Oil

o Roasted Sesame Oil

o Flaxseed Oil

o Flavored Oils

Remember, oil is not your enemy when it comes to healthy eating. These are actually essential to the functions if your body and brain. They also help the body absorb vitamins A, D, E and K. Aside from that, they can also add extra flavor and depth to your dishes—so it all boils down to choosing the right ones.

- Quinoa is another pantry staple. Often referred to as the "miracle" grain, this is versatile and can be used for breakfast, lunch or dinner. It can be prepared sweet or savory—depending on your taste. If you're looking for an alternative to white rice, this is a great option to try.

- Dried fruit preserves are also great to keep in your pantry. These serve as great breakfast toppings, especially for yogurt. You can also use them in baking bread or to add flavors to your regular sandwiches.

- Do avoid purchasing bagged potato chips, making your own is better and healthier. The best bit is that homemade chips take less than hour to put together and you can flavor them in any way you like as well. This wouldn't contain trans fats so you can be certain that you're having a healthy snack. Another alternative? Sweet potato and banana chips.

These are just a few tips you can use for putting together a grocery list. Remember, always opt for fresh and organic. The more basic it is the better, too!

Conclusion

I'd like to thank you and congratulate you for transiting my lines from start to finish.

I hope this book was able to help you to better understand what Meal Prep , how to lose weight effectively.

The next step is to give the program a try and switch to the recipes provided here. Truth is, in doing so, there's really nothing for you to lose other than a bit of excess weight. We can keep telling you how great this program is when it comes to improving your health, but nothing beats actually experiencing it for yourself.

I wish you the best of luck!

BONUS CONTENT

Dash Diet Cookbook
Breakfast Recipes

French Toast

Calories 229

Total Carbohydrate 25 g

Saturated fat 2.7 g

Total Fat 11 g

Sodium 479 mg

Protein 8 g

Number of Servings: 2

Ingredients:

- 2 egg whites

- 4 slices whole wheat bread

- 1 whole egg

- ½ tsp. pure vanilla extract

- ½ cup unsweetened almond milk

- ¼ tsp. ground cinnamon

- 1/8 tsp. ground nutmeg

- Olive oil cooking spray

- ¼ tsp. brown sugar

For garnish

- pure maple syrup

- fresh fruit slices

- yogurt

Directions:

➤ Beat the egg whites with the egg in a large bowl. Add the almond milk, brown sugar, cinnamon, nutmeg, and vanilla extract. Mix well.

➤ Place one slice of bread into the mixture and ensure the slice is coated completely.

➤ While the slice is soaking, place a non-stick skillet over medium flame and spray with some olive oil.

➤ Remove the soaked slice of bread and place in the hot pan. Place the second slice in the egg mixture and allow to soak.

➢ Cook the French toast for about 2 minutes per side, or until browned all over. Transfer to a platter and cook the second slice.

➢ Once both pieces of French toast are ready, serve right away. This is best served with maple syrup or yogurt and fresh fruit on top.

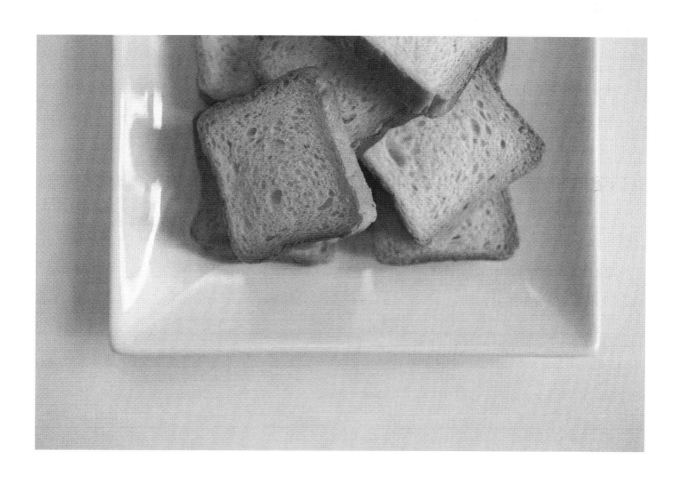

Whole Wheat Hotcakes

Calories 340

Total Carbohydrate 72 g

Saturated fat 0.4 g

Total Fat 2.5 g

Sodium 2 mg

Protein 13 g

Number of Servings: 2-4 servings

Ingredients:

- 1 cup white whole wheat flour

- 1 egg

- 6 tablespoons buttermilk powder

- ¼ cup ground flaxseed

- 1 teaspoon baking powder

- 1 teaspoon baking soda

- ½ teaspoon ground cinnamon

- 2 tablespoons canola oil

- 1 ½ cup water

- Pinch of salt

Directions:

➢ In a large mixing bowl, combine the baking powder, flour, baking soda, buttermilk powder, flaxseed, and cinnamon. Beat the egg. Stir in the oil and water.

➢ Add the flour mixture and whisk. Let it sit for 5 minutes.

➤ Heat a griddle and coat with cooking spray. Ladle equal portions of batter onto the griddle. Cook for 2 minutes or until browned on the sides and bubbles start to form on top.

➤ Flip on the other side and cook for 2 minutes.

➤ Repeat steps with the other pancakes. Serve.

Cheesy Egg and Spinach on Wheat Toast

Calories 351

Total Carbohydrate 25.4 g

Saturated fat 9.8 g

Total Fat 23.6 g

Sodium 209mg

Protein 11.1g

Number of Servings: 2

Ingredients:

- 2 slices whole wheat bread

- 3 egg whites, beaten

- ¾ cup baby spinach

- 2 tomato slices

- 1 ½ tsp. brown mustard

- 2 thin slices low fat cheddar cheese

- 2 tsp. extra virgin olive oil

- Black pepper

Directions:

➢ Set the oven to 400 degrees F to preheat.

➢ Place a non-stick pan over medium flame and heat through. Once hot, add the olive oil and swirl to coat.

➢ Add the egg whites and scramble until cooked to a desired consistency. Then, add the spinach and sprinkle in some pepper. Stir well.

➢ Spread the brown mustard on one side of each slice of bread. Then, add the tomato slices on top, followed by the scrambled egg whites.

➢ Add the cheese on top, then place the slices on a baking sheet. Bake for 2 minutes or until the cheese melts and the bread is lightly toasted.

➢ Transfer to a serving plate and serve right away.

Nutty Banana Pancakes

Calories 227

Total Carbohydrate 30.1 g

Saturated fat 1.4 g

Total Fat 9.9 g

Sodium 287 mg

Protein 6.3 g

Number of Servings: 3

Ingredients:

- 2 egg whites

- 1 banana, mashed

- 1 tsp. baking powder

- ½ cup whole wheat flour

- 1 tsp. coconut oil, melted

- ½ tsp. pure vanilla extract

- Ground cinnamon, to taste

- 1 Tbsp. walnuts, finely chopped

Directions:

➢ Combine all the dry ingredients in a mixing bowl, then create a pit in the center.

➢ Whisk the egg whites and milk in a separate bowl, then add the vanilla extract and mix well. Mash in the banana then stir in the coconut oil and mix well.

➢ Combine the dry and wet ingredients until lumpy smooth. Do not over-mix as the pancakes will turn out tough.

➢ Place a pancake griddle over medium flame and heat through. Once hot, add a bit of oil and swirl to coat.

➢ Cook the pancakes until firm, about 1 minute per side, then place on a platter. Best served warm.